SYMPOSIUM

JOSHUA GRAY

Symposium
Copyright © 2016 Joshua Gray

ISBN-13: 978-1523765218

Cover art © Public domain from NASA
Bio portrait © Rebecca Venn
Cover Design © 2016 Red Dashboard LLC Publications

Published by
Red Dashboard LLC Publishing
Princeton NJ 08540
www.reddashboard.com

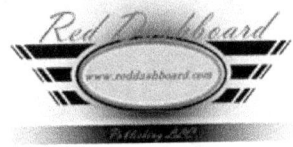

For Ketaki

Acknowlegements

These poems first appeared in the following journals:

"I Am Gilgamesh": MO: *Writings from the River*
"Garden": *FreeXpression*
"The Many Goodbyes": *Poesia*
"Quilting": *Front Range Review*
"Ass Pleasure", "Hallway Painting": *Poets and Artists*
"Results Received": *VerseWright*
"Awaiting The Cure", "Sestina For Turning Forty": *Survivors Review*
"Melancholy": *Jujubes*
"The Finish Off": *iArtistas*
"Symbiote": *Z-Composition*

I am especially thankful to the following people and medical centers. They are, perhaps literally, life savers.

Lisa Kaufman, MD and Todd E. Perkins, MD who suspected and confirmed Melanoma. Malini Devanandan, MD who told me four years later those fleabites were actually moles, and my mother and step-father for the long and unexpected stay.

Stephen Evans, MD, Anne McArdle APRN, Michael Atkins, MD and Kellie Parks, APRN at Georgetown University Hospital's Department of General Surgery and Vince Lombardi Cancer Center.

Jason Chesney, MD, PhD and the Brown Cancer Center at the University of Louisville Medical Center.

The music of Jenny Bruce and Krishna Das for sustaining me through very difficult times, and my wife Ketaki, to whom this book is dedicated, for being my rock. For everything.

Table of Contents

Attendees *3*
The Many Goodbyes *4*
Quilting *6*
A Typical Life Until *8*
Gold Blood, Blood Gold *10*
Déjà vu *12*
Reentry *13*

Opening Remarks *15*
I Am Gilgamesh *16*

First Speaker (Diagnosis/Surgery) *19*
Results Received *20*
Results, Stage Three *22*
Going Under Anesthesia *23*
Awaiting The Cure *24*
Ass Pleasure *26*
Hallway Painting *28*
Ultraviolet *30*
Sestina for Turning Forty *33*
Home From the Hospital *35*

Keynote Address (Treatment) *39*
On The Way, A Blessing *40*
Back At Ground Zero *41*
Fool *44*
Butterfly Effect *46*
Trial *48*
Relating the Day *50*
Dream Not Of Death *52*
Melancholy *54*
Narcissism *56*
The Finish Off *57*
Symbiote *59*

Closing Remarks *63*
Garden *64*

ATTENDEES

The Many Goodbyes

She smelled It and stared
into the white robe at a stain
reflection, and It was sour.
Anger penetrated the hour
as the fear closed in, as the pain
turned, worsened, and dared

to divide their yoke.
He touched It afterwards
and before the wake waned.
At last open blinds were gained;
written words teamed towards
the past as the rage chose to choke

his support. And even I –
I tasted It when I heard the blow
of that speedy disease. In the end
I was left aloof, alone, to spend
all of It, while the circles would show
up to stir their lost goodbye.

Pancreatic cancer accounts for about 3% of all cancers in the US, and accounts for about 7% of cancer deaths. ~ American Cancer Society

Pancreatic cancer is aggressive with few symptoms until the cancer is advanced. – WebMD

Quilting

Your life is a quilt. You weave the wonders
of Appalachia into the mundane mid-west.
You will talk of Hinduism
and in the same breath remind us of the Quakers.

You speak of how the Indians use their cold ashes
to clean the plates they eat off of,
and we laugh at your rejection of a soap
because it changes color.

You tossed that soap out
not as an invalidation of us, but because
that patch we've picked for you
doesn't flow in your design.

What a reservoir of knowledge
you have, bits of fabric sewn
into our unsuspecting hearts. We now know
if the glacier or the river formed the valley.

But the Bhutanese valleys
are another thing. You have declared
Bhutan heaven on earth,
because it is so hard to get to. Too hard.

And yet, your resourcefulness
has gotten you there. Is Heaven
everything you expected it to be,
with its gross national happiness?

You left behind your quilt.
Before your plane could rise above us,

your quilt expanded to cover more
than you ever thought possible.

How beautiful it is, how it touches
the crafts only our dreams create.
It was well worth the artistry of effort.
Don't forget to send a postcard.

In the case of my mother-in-law, from diagnosis of pancreatic cancer to
her passing was a period of about ten weeks.

A Typical Life Until

She drove home, alone and deep
within her periodic tables.
She never stopped
paying attention to the asphalt
and the swarming five o'clockers.

A blaring horn brought
her to the old blue minivan,
it's pollen-stained windshield,
the empty plastic bottle
bumping into her ankles.

The screeching brakes beside her
did no good. Her left arm flung
toward the gears; her leg pinned
itself into the right, her head hit
by something else entirely.

Shock descended ~ found her
fastened between her door
and a warm ray of sunshine~
and enveloped her pain, softening it
into weightless humid air.

Mammography misses about 16 percent of breast cancers. Depending on certain factors (such as breast density) mammography may miss nearly 30 percent of breast cancers. ~ Susan G Komen/komen.org

Besides skin cancer [Gray's italics], breast cancer is the most commonly diagnosed cancer among American women.
– breastcancer.org

Gold Blood, Blood Gold

No one thought it could be. Once

the doctors pinned her bone-sand leg
and x-rayed her frayed ribs,
they discovered stage four Breast, despite
that mammogram which spoke nada.

Better call hospice, but *hell no*,
and so she beat red beets to blood,
and got rich off gold Turmeric.
She drank her pills and wore her wig.

Her appetite escaped
her teeth and trap, supper the taste
of cardboard. Constant puja to Durga.
She returned to work, earning life its fullest

to fool those that grew fast as
Eucalyptus. Red smudges on scans
shrank, so she kept her focus.
From spins to moons to orbits,

to not one red dot. No one thought
it could be.

Laboratory tests have found that turmeric interferes with many critical molecular pathways that cause the growth and spread of cancer...A number of lab studies have found that curcumin [the active ingredient in Turmeric] kills cancer cells and prevents growth of cells that survive. It is also found to shrink tumors and prevent some cancers in laboratory animals. – turmericforhealth.com

Some breakthrough studies have shown that the same characteristics in beets – which help athletes perform better – help cancer patients reverse their condition. The link between oxygen and cancer is well known and beets can increase oxygen, within the blood, by 400 percent while helping to eliminate waste products. – naturalhealth365.com

Deja Vu

He slipped through the side door
and cursed the hard, cracked chair
in which he sat.

Approximately **14.0 percent** of men will be diagnosed with prostate
cancer at some point during their lifetime, based on 2010-2012 data. –
Surveillance, Epidemiology, and End Results Program (SEER), National
Cancer Institute

Reentry

Father, do not fall
from the heavens as if
you skydive
with no chute.

You fall fast and flail arms.

But it's far better to flex
tissue as you bend
the tight barrier
between us.

The number of [Prostate Cancer] deaths was 21.4 per 100,000 men per year. These rates are age-adjusted and based on 2008-2012 cases and deaths. ~ SEER, National Cancer Institute

Opening Remarks

I Am Gilgamesh

(Prologue)

I built walls and not one gets through.
I am perfect.

(Enkido)

Barbaric-born,
He never did care for this world.
But some harlot lured him forth,
Clothed and offered as my first-born.
I take no blame for his psychosis.

(Humbaba)

Together we tackle the cause,
A lone enigma we cannot
See, hear, touch, but a watchman no
Less, for the large and darkened woods

(Death)

Lurk too close. Strength weakens
When shadowed. Love set aside,
I lose desire for his goodwill.
I feel my soul tire with age

(Quest)

As I reach this crisis sooner.
I search for a plan,
A plan to move like the gods.
Important. Someone. Alive,

(Flood)

Instead of when I almost drowned
Under pressure of weathered life,
A bath among the dead.
In drew Noah with the sun,

(Return)

Its shining arms reached down to grab
My thoughts like a lost tablet
Found, wound me up like an instrument,
For I am King.

FIRST SPEAKER
DIAGNOSIS/SURGERY

Results Received

I do not need the dark gray duvet
hovering high above
to remind me this is not
the first storm to come today.
I woke up expecting sunny skies,
passing puffs of clouds
just a memory
of potential disaster. But one dim cloud
had the nerve to dampen
the sunniest point of my compass.
The sky turned overcast gently.
Maybe I marched out into it
because I had to meet it head on.
Thunder never forced its way
into my deaf ears; lightning never gripped
my eyeglasses. Occasional drops
squeezed my shirt collar, or slapped my knee.
There was no one near me
to feel the weight of my Adam's Apple
dropping ever so slightly down my throat.
But I was in it nonetheless,
the storm came unannounced.
My socks were soaked.
It wasn't until after I jumped
from the tempest outside
back into the dry house
that I noticed how soaked I was.
Clothes clung to my body
as I desperately tried to remove them.
I grabbed a dry towel and gave it water
by passing it over my body,
sighing all the while. Now, as I lie
on my couch exhausted, looking out the window,
waiting for a new storm I know is coming,
I wonder how much

I will experience the sensations
as they come over me,
notice that I am getting drenched, or at least
notice when I need to run ~
dodging each drop as it free falls above me ~
into the security of a drained home.

Melanoma rates doubled between 1982 and 2011 ~ Center for Disease
Control (CDC)

This year [2015], an estimated 137,000 Americans will be diagnosed with
melanoma. ~ Melanoma Research Foundation

Going Under Anesthesia

I'm rolled in on a bed. Fingers and palms lower the handrails.
Narrow bed next to me.

Scoot over.

Lying on the narrow bed, left arm placed on foam extension.
Right upper arm under pressure, my heavy pulse. Then release.
Numbers announced.

'Is that good?'

Very good.

Thermometer swiped across my forehead, cheek.
Trouble on the right. I look –
Arm foam extension not there.

Can you jerk it free?

There.

Right arm placed like I'm being crucified.
One black strap over my legs.

Are you allergic to any medication?

'No.'

Two black straps over my legs.

Any circulation problems?

'No.'

Plastic inserted into my nostrils.

How's that?

'Okay.'

Body heavy, relaxes. Eyesight blurs...

'Oh. Cooool.

See you guys when I wake up.'

Eyelids drop, reopen.

'Feels like the old college days.'

Laughs heard. Eyes shut. Blackness.

A hospital bed is a parked taxi with the meter running.
~ Groucho Marx

Awaiting The Cure

Someday a specialist
won't have to dig a hole
in my foot;
no plastic surgeon
will need to fill the hole
with a speck of skin
from my thigh;
there will be a time
when my groin isn't sliced open
to find a node,
or worse, a train
of nodes ~ no resident will staple
my open wound, along with
my gentle spirit ~
but that day will come
after the soul has left this body:
nobody
has led the way, though the world is full
of those who've tried;
and while the world waits
I fight
to claim my skin,
awaiting the cure
to creep into the glass slide, the petri dish,
the arms of Everyman.

More than 40 years after the war on cancer was declared, we have spent billions fighting the good fight. The National Cancer Institute has spent some $90 billion on research and treatment during that time...It's true there have been small declines in some common cancers since the early 1990s...And the fall in the cancer death rate — by approximately 1 percent a year since 1990 — has been slightly more impressive. Still, that's hardly cause for celebration. Cancer's role in one out of every four deaths in this country remains a haunting statistic...Simply put, we have not adequately channeled our scientific know-how, funding, and energy into a full exploration of the one path certain to save lives: prevention...When I look at NCI's budget request for fiscal year 2012, I'm deeply disappointed, though past experience tells me I shouldn't be surprised. It is business as usual at the nation's foremost cancer research establishment. More than $2 billion is requested for basic research into the mechanism and causes of cancer. Another $1.3 billion is requested for treatment. And cancer prevention and control? It gets $232 million altogether.

~ Dr. Margaret Cuomo, author of *A World Without Cancer*

Ass Pleasure

I admit to the twinge
of guilt while I stared
at the nurse's ass
as she justly stood
outside my room
communicating
with her computer.
All day I coveted
that ass with my wife
right beside me,
holding my hand.
She wasn't even my nurse,
but the charge nurse,
the head honcho.
Yet my eyes never left
her been-around bell curves.
She was no stereotype
of the cute nurse,
not the way my nurse
fit the image.
But my nurse had no ass.
And there was something
about the charge nurse's ass
from under
those sky blue
slightly ruffled
loosely fitted
street pants
that drew my eyes
away
from my wife.

Nurses are often required to work long shifts. But in a number of cases, nurses must work back-to-back or extended shifts, risking fatigue that could result in medical mistakes...A 2012 study published in *Health Affairs* found that the longer the shifts for hospital nurses, the higher the levels of burnout and patient dissatisfaction...And a 2014 study in the *American Journal of Critical Care* found that nurses impaired by fatigue, loss of sleep, daytime sleepiness and an inability to recover between shifts are more likely than well-rested nurses to report decision regret, a negative cognitive emotion that occurs when the actual outcome differs from the desired or expected outcome.
~ Beckers Hospital Review

There is no on-the-job training for nurses. ~ Bureau of Labor Statistics

Hallway Painting

For days I looked at it outside my hospital room,
screwed on the wall:
a group of amber trees waved in the northwest wind,
stretching themselves into a swirl
of ivory intention.

If I had been high on mushrooms, or a paper square,
I would have thought the trees were people
being pulled skyward like rubber stakes
into the torque of a tornado or hurricane,
with the eye patiently black, dark, listlessly silent.

But I was not high. There was no hurricane.
The trees were being whisked into some other world,
which eased them from their groundings
and brought them through
the tunnel of time.

When I was able
to hobble out into the hallway, I discovered
my own treachery: the trees
were just the outermost petal of a flower,
the black center of the tunnel simply a landing pad
for a passing butterfly.

On the Oncology floor at Georgetown University Hospital in Washington DC, whenever a patient dies the nurses hang a butterfly on their door.

Ultraviolet

1.

The sun stares
unblinkingly
into my skin.

The sun is a large proton,
a cobalt lead ball
lit in flames.

It is an eye, the dark
watchman
of middle earth.

It is a serial killer that cuts
us while we listen
to the poetry of waves.

2.

He's never prayed
to God, but believes
they understand each other.

She can take him before
he's ready, after his suffering,
as long as the sun stays employed.

For the sun warms lake water
filled with sky and provides food
to the forest green ferns.

It rises to high noon

so the blind
mole can find its way.

Every evening the sun
entertains us with rich hues
stroked along its blue canvas,

and flashes its spotlight
so the small lizards can crawl
across our cut grass at night.

That's all great, he tells her,
just make sure of its omnipresence
for my children when I'm gone.

3.

Too bad the sunspots are malignant,
and no oncologist exists in space
to save the sun from its own black hole.

More than 90 percent of melanoma skin cancers are due to skin cell damage from ultraviolet (UV) radiation exposure. ~ CDC

Sestina For Turning Forty

My big day barely over, my body
believed I should act my age.
I stared at the mushroomed mole
resting below my toes. It stung. It itched.
After my biopsy, the pain kicked in.
Restful nights lost their way.

Melanoma wandered through the entranceway
of my stressed-out and worn-down body,
found a warm cozy place, and settled in.
I thanked the sky for the modern age
of medicine; even as each day passed, I itched
for a time when no one spoke of the mole.

But my friends, they only discussed the mole.
Of course, I learned the best way
to play the game was to beat every itch
I had to stay still when the doorbell rang. Everybody
had my back, after all. Perhaps my age
created this reclusive stage I was in.

Three summers of family cares and cancer was in:
pancreas, breast, and now skin. Who was the mole
hiding within, and at what young age
does a crook's life begin? Jokes were the way
to lighten my mood ~ my body,
though bruised, retained a joyful itch.

The staples from my surgery started to itch.
My back was sore from the hard bed I was in.
The best times meant friends ~ the worst, nobody.
I laughed alone in the darkness of moles.
The hospital food was horrendous ~ no curds and whey
for me. Nutrition and medicine have their separate ages.

When I finally went home, a well-aged
wine was opened. I itched
for the outdoors, a good way
to feel whole again. But I stayed in;
I was too broken. I didn't search for moles.
I claimed my own skin. It was mine. It was my body.

That's the way my forties began. I was in over my head.
One itch led to another. One mole made me insane.
I only have one body, after all, and it changes with age.

Aging is the single biggest risk factor for developing cancer. ~ Cancer.net

Home From The Hospital

If ever there were a day to breathe crisp air,
where the rolling green Appalachians soothe me
or the spiked white Himalayans own me,
that day would be this day.

If ever there were a day where I can roll back
and have a cold drink with a warm friend
who gives me the gift of my heartiest laugh,
that day would be this day.

If ever there were a day that challenges me
with a soft hand on my hard shoulder,
the way a poem discovers me on its birthday,
that would be this day.

This day is a ripe day, the right way
to turn from rotten and callous times, when
I've forgotten such a day that must begin
this day.

That first hopeful optimistic day.
That.

KEYNOTE SPEAKER TREATMENT

On The Way, A Blessing

The blue phoenix flew close,
landed among the clutter of dry grass,
dropped his head to a bow.

Melanoma patients are told that they can be considered survivors when
they've gone five years with no evidence of disease (NED). I went four.

Back To Ground Zero

-- For Anne

The dark brown wooden mammoth
of a desk housed its pool of low wagers.
The printer sang off key
while the receptionist handed a clipboard
full of mundane forms, and a pen,
to her latest victim of somber anxiety.

A tall pale-skinned woman left
her chair and walked up to the refreshment table,
removed a styrofoam cup,
poured her black water, her way-too-much sugar
and non-dairy creamer, then nervously took her seat.

My wife flipped through another old magazine.
as my mother turned to her smartphone
and scrolled through e-mails.

The receptionist walked around
the desk and opened the door
to the administrative offices
but did not walked into it.
She then returned to her seat, as if
there was no reason why she moved about.

A nurse walked up the hallway
and called a name. An old man got up
and followed her, cane employed,
past the bathrooms, and into the nest
of sterile rooms.
The elevator opened its doors with a ding
and people exchanged places.

My mother laughed at what
she read, and many eyes turned,
jealous they had nothing
to laugh about.

The receptionist handed over
another clipboard. Another name
was called, and a young woman
with a full head of hair meandered off.
A team of ducklings followed.
I did not hear the elevator door,

but there she was, standing before me,
dressed in bleach, her loose-knit wrap
over her shoulders, curly dark hair
under her flimsy nurse's hat.
Four years later, she looked the same,

My wife and I stood to greet her,
my mother followed suit, aware
of who she must be.

We smiled and thanked her,
told her we'd see her soon,
then let her go clock in.

We never saw her again.
My name was never called.

in-transit metastasis (in-TRAN-zit meh-TAS-tuh-sis):
A type of metastasis in which skin cancer spreads through a lymph vessel and begins to grow more than 2 centimeters away from the primary tumor but before it reaches the nearest lymph node. – NCI

In-transit metastases...occur shortly (mean, 16 months) after definitive treatment of the primary melanoma in 10% of patients.
~ cancernetwork.com

The management of in-transit metastases is challenging, since the treatments and extent of disease vary greatly based on the number, depth, location, and distribution of lesions, and on their biological behavior. – cancernetwork.com

A Fool's Gift

These malignant cells breast stroking
within my dark corridors
play the fool. The noise grates.
Snipers attack.

They are my subordinates.
They are unworthy to survive
their own sacrifice because they can't play nice.
But the most favored guest at supper
is the clown.

They only exist to say how
I'm the fool, just the jester
creating an iamb grasping for a spondee
in a pyrrhic's stead.

I do not like this feeling of fatigue,
or the infectious low-lifes luring
me into cellular genocide.

I thank the knife. I thank
this wise-up call along the highways
of my leg. Self-neglect casted me
to play the fool.

Clown: Good madonna, why mournest thou?
Olivia: Good fool, for my brother's death.
Clown: I think his soul is in hell, madonna.
Olivia: I know his soul is in heaven, fool.
Clown:The more fool, madonna, to mourn for your brother's
	soul being in heaven.
 ~Twelfth Night, Act I Scene V

This book will serve as a revelation for those who are sufficiently open-minded to consider the possibility that cancer and other debilitating illnesses are not actual diseases, but desperate and final attempts by the body to stay alive for as long as circumstances permit.

It will perhaps astound you to learn that a person who is afflicted with the main causes of cancer (which constitute the real illness) would most likely die quickly unless he actually grew cancer cells. In this work, I provide evidence to this effect.

I further claim that cancer will only occur after all other defense or healing mechanisms in the body have failed.

~ Andreas Moritz, author of *Cancer is not a Disease - It's a Survival Mechanism*

Butterfly Effect

The birth of a butterfly signals another life
lost to metastases. Every elegant monarch
resting on the leaf of a turning maple is the spirit
of a mother, a brother, another friend.

With each flap of its bright wing,
the monarch alters the delicate course
of our lives. Every breath it takes is full
of a departed soul.

A feathered beast can lose its valor.
The eagle is fragile and flees into the forest
whenever it's been forgotten.

But the eagle will always soar into the wind
to carry us along
the frayed path of a butterfly.

The man who has no imagination has no wings.
~ Muhammad Ali

Trial

The silent dark deep
tunnels surround a large
still swimming pool.
Nothing moves within its trap.
The air I break fails to scream.

I've seen the natives,
victims of my own invasion.

I am their death,
should the white king fall.
I move from square to square unnoticed.

They've noticed me.

They hear my featherweight feet
on the cold damp floor.
and feel the air cool
as I pass by.

I start to sweat through my black cloth
as they light lanterns and quicken their pace.

I find the way
out of my dark, deep tunnel and rush
into the pool, crashing
its immense peace.

One new therapy for Melanoma is a combination of Ipilimumab and Nivolumab. Cancer cells have a coating on them that essentially keeps them invisible from the immune system. Ipilimumab is an immune-booster, and Nivolumab is an anti-PD1, which breaks the cancer cell coating, allowing the immune system to identify and attack them.

Relating The Day

I ordered
a smoked calf,
cut up. But

in the box
lived a live
giant chicken.

I hid it
in the kitchen
away from

the vegetarian.
I mean you.
But the bird

was killing the
cookhouse and you
came back home

so I moved
it to the barn
but not before

falling deep
into a bucket
of shit.

I was on the extended dosage trial of the Ippi/Anti-PD1 combo. The side effects of this treatment that I experienced include dry mouth, itching, nausea, liver enzyme count that increased ten times the normal range, and apparently, weird dreams.

Dream Not Of Death

Your truth is trapped inside its past. The future may be lying.
Dream of joy in sorrow but never while you sleep.
Do not fight the glare of death. Fear the state of dying.

How the day can twist and flow, as you sit here sighing.
These moments bear tomorrow and often break or weep.
Your truth is trapped inside its past. The future may be lying.

To be a man is difficult with aging parents prying;
It's best to set the stage that earns your soul its keep.
Do not fight the glare of death. Fear the state of dying.

Another life in a distant time may be far less trying;
The one you borrowed now will sting you as it seeps.
Your truth is trapped inside its past. The future may be lying.

As you lie in bed at night tired from all that crying ~
For sleep is daily practice for a grimmer reap ~
Do not fight the glare of death. Fear the state of dying.

The fortune tellers read your dreams, but reading isn't buying.
A book of lonely thoughts commands itself to speak.
Your truth is trapped inside its past. The future may be lying.
Do not fight the glare of death. Fear the state of dying.

Approximately 50% of melanoma patients' tumor tissue tests positive for this genetic mutation [BRAF]. A mutated BRAF accelerates tumor cell growth and this change can increase the growth and spread of cancer cells. – Melanoma International Foundation

BRAF (B-RAF) treatment is considered a last resort/end-of-life attempt to extend a patient's life by a couple years.

Melancholy

This morning the waiting room is full
of empty chairs. Someone sits and speaks
to no one I can see. The TV
I rarely watch mutely wears a cable
news show telling us how we will all die.

The harp player has left
her instrument, wrapped in its soft red bag,
leaning against the sterile wall.
I have always wanted to thank her for her service,
But my blue shin cannot match her Greensleeves.

The painter is not here today. His table holds
nothing but brochures on a bright sky.
He often paints flowers, thin as his hair, and invites others
to join him in a voice that radiates from his gray beard.
But even he is silent.

My wife had to work today. She could not come
to sit in that corner and solve
yet another puzzle, spread on a square table.
I cannot leave her
to go measure precisely how sick I am.

Go into the arts. I'm not kidding. The arts are not a way to make a living. They are a very human way of making life more bearable. Practicing an art, no matter how well or badly, is a way to make your soul grow, for heaven's sake. Sing in the shower. Dance to the radio. Tell stories. Write a poem to a friend, even a lousy poem. Do it as well as you possibly can. You will get an enormous reward. You will have created something. - Kurt Vonnegut

Narcissism

So what if
I'm late. I fell
through
my eyes, landed
under my skin.

What does it mean to be an oncologist? It means that you get to sit in at a moment of another person's life that is so hyper-acute, and not just because they're medically ill. It's also a moment of hope and expectation and concern.

~ Siddhartha Mukherjee, Pulitzer Prize winner for *The Emperor of All Maladies: A Biography of Cancer*

The Finish Off

After the white coats went their merry way,
I decided to kill Cerberus myself. He growled
as I drew near, unveiling those ivory teeth.

I bit down hard on my chewing gum,
and sprayed fragrant oil onto each foaming head
of the dusty gray dog. The scent soured his noses,
and he dropped his heads and tucked in his tail.

Then I pulled out the *Eau de Légumes Pourris*
and threw it in his faces. He stepped back
and yelped, fur turning blood red,
so I spit my gum onto one of his snouts,
laughed at his grand ol' cinnamon mole.

Finally, I drenched him with the extra oxygen
that surrounded me. His heads shrunk
like bubble gum bubbles losing air. His red fur
went as pale as those old white coats,
and the three-headed dog turned so sterile
it seemed he had taken off, tail clenching belly,
at the utter agony of joy.

There are many alternative topical medicines one can put on their Melanoma moles. I chose to go with Frankincense oil, Neem Oil and Hydrogen Peroxide, to varied successes.

Symbiote

She doesn't give you Herpes.

                        Instead, she dons
a loosely-fitted spaghetti-strapped red dress,
and begins on your shin. She lowers
to cover the ankle, creeps onto the knee
and anchors herself. It is the only time
her weight is felt.

With increased momentum, she moves in
over the stomach, the chest, the back.
She bruises your neck. As you sleep,
she french kisses your open mouth.

When you wake up, you discover
she's even found the insides
of your elbows. You do not fail to notice
she took some time on your hips.

The only way to free yourself
is to allow your emotions
to possess you.

But she doesn't give you Herpes ~
you give it to yourself.

[T-VEC] is a genetically modified herpes simplex virus. Scientists modified it so that when it gets into cells, it can grow and multiply in cancer cells but not in healthy cells. It works by being administered directly into the cancer cell and then as it multiplies, it busts open the cell wall and the cancer cell dies. Also, it has on the back end, the granulocyte-macrophage colony-stimulating factor (GM-CSF), which stimulates the immune system. So the idea is that if you deliver it right to the cancer cell, it can help the body memorize the proteins that part of that cancer cell [sic] and then other areas of melanoma might shrink in the course of giving this product. ~ Frances Collichio MD, University of North Carolina School of Medicine (Chapel Hill) and one of the study authors

After more than nine years of oncologists administering the T-VEC/Herpes treatment in clinical trial settings, there have been two known cases of patients breaking out into an allergic reaction in the form of a reddish full body rash. I was one of them.

Closing Remarks

Garden

I am determined to seed my garden.
Early Spring, lettuce and green leaf
Plants need planting. I'm too young
For the child my wife carries. The last frost
Of bedroom's winter came too late.

I am tempted to cede my garden.
Early summer, pests munch and kill
The plants I planted. The pest that threatens
My child we call some acronym for
Hope and ignorance: a serpent's sweet fruit.

THE IMPORTANCE OF POETRY

Poetry is the oldest form of written language that is still used today. It communicates our strongest emotions and our deepest thoughts. So many people do not read poetry because they do not understand it, but they do not understand it because they do not read it. If you don't practice piano you won't be able to play — the same principle applies to poetry. It can open up an entire universe if you only allow it to; it is the divine language.

Poet's Statement:

Music is the driving force in my poetry. It dictates how characters, themes, voice, and other important aspects of the craft are developed. There are so many ways in which music can play a part, and each poem has a different balance of weights as the ones before. The beauty and joy in my writing is finding that balance. I am inspired by both classical and modern poets who value music as much as I do.

Much of my poetry centers around understanding the human condition. I enjoy internal dialogues between aspects of a single character as well as open dialogues in pursuit of stronger relationships and clearer understandings at a universal level.

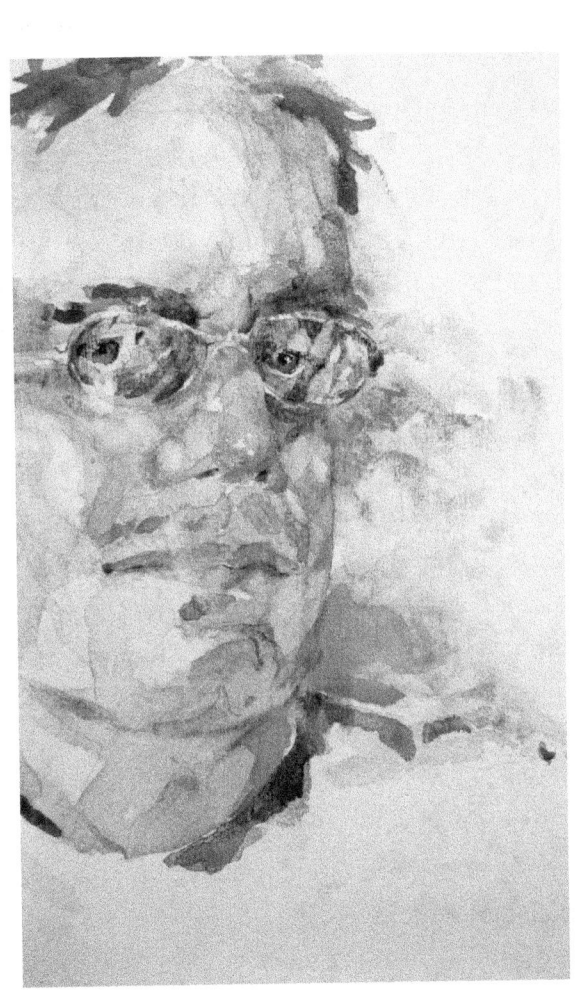

ABOUT THE AUTHOR

Joshua Gray was born in the mountains of rural Northern Virginia, outside Washington DC. He grew up in Alexandria VA, two miles from the nation's capital and spent most of his adult life in the suburbs of the city. But he never lost his love for the mountains: he attended Warren Wilson College in the mountains of western North Carolina, and lived in the Western Ghats mountains in Kodaikanal, Tamil Nadu, India from 2012-2014. He now lives in eastern Kentucky with his wife and two sons.

He has been published in many journals, including *Poets and Artists, Mipoesias, Blind Man's Rainbow, Front Range Review, Iconoclast, Zouch Magazine* and many others. His poetry has been nominated for Best of the Net, nominated for a Pushcart Prize, and featured on Verse Daily's Web Weekly section. For two years he was the DC Poetry Examiner for Examiner.com where he wrote reviews of poetry collections by local poets as well as articles on the local poetry scene. He is active on Twitter, Facebook, StumbleUpon and many other social media sites.

His first book *Beowulf: A Verse adaptation With Young Readers In Mind* was written for his oldest son when he was six, but as the title implies, it can be enjoyed by an older audience, including adults. His book-length poem *Principles of Belonging* is based on true stories about his parents and parents-in-law, and is written using many different poetry forms, including some modernized ancient forms. His chapbook *Mera Bharat* is a collection of poems based on his experiences in India, and was published in 2014. In 2015 he published *Steel Cut Oats*, a collection of poems that honor the traditions of food from a cultural standpoint, rejecting the modern processed and unhealthy food industry.

www.reddashboard.com

www.ingramcontent.com/pod-product-compliance
Lightning Source LLC
Chambersburg PA
CBHW062102280526
45788CB00003B/1315